Clean Eating: Detox Diet:

Clean Food & Plant Based Diet; Detox Cleanse Diet to Lose Belly Fat & Increase Energy

Emma Rose

Clean Eating Guide

Lose Weight Quickly, Achieve Optimal Health and Feel Energized with Clean Eating for Busy Families and Clean Eating Recipes

Emma Rose

Table of Contents

Introduction

I want to thank you and congratulate you for purchasing the book, *"**Clean Eating Guide**: Lose Weight Quickly, Achieve Optimal Health and Feel Energized with Clean Eating For Busy Families and Clean Eating Recipes"*.

This book contains proven steps and strategies on how to lose weight, have more energy, and stay healthy using the principles of clean eating.

There are so many different kinds of diet programs and products available in the market today and all you need to do is choose the one that you think will work best for you. If you do not want to try new products that helps you lose weight and boosts your energy, you should stick to something more basic and natural such as clean eating.

In this book, you will learn everything you need to know about clean eating. It is important to find out everything you can about this type of diet before you incorporate it in your lifestyle. You will learn about the benefits and principles of clean eating and some useful tips that can help you along the way. This book also includes some easy recipes that promote clean eating.

Thanks again for purchasing this book, I hope you enjoy it! Please take some time to stop by and LIKE our Facebook page:

https://www.facebook.com/joypublishing

With gratitude,

Emma Rose

Chapter 1

What Is Clean Eating?

You have probably come across the term 'clean eating' but you are still not familiar about its exact meaning. This is being used by people who work in the health and fitness industry such as personal trainers ad dietitians. People who are health conscious and workout fanatic also often use this word. Does it have something to do with cleaning the food before eating or cooking? Or maybe it has something to do with the kind of food that you eat.

The loose definition of clean eating is eating food in its most natural state. These days, people are starting to pay more attention to the kinds of food that they eat and how these foods are made. They take note of the food's ingredients and make sure that the food product only contains all natural ingredients.

The term clean eating first came out in the 1990s. Today, it is still being used by health conscious individuals from different backgrounds and culture to refer to the kind of all natural diet that they have. The definition of clean eating can vary from person to person. Some define clean eating as eating mostly fruits and vegetables while others define it as not eating anything artificial. You will find out more about these things as you read this book.

What Clean Eating is not?

If you think clean eating is another diet program, like the South Beach diet or Paleo diet, you are wrong because clean eating is a way of life. It also does not follow any strict rules about what food group to eat and not to eat, how many calories you should consume in a meal, and so on. This is the most basic way of healthy eating that promotes weight loss and boost energy.

Everybody can do this, even those who are not trying to lose weight.

Clean eating will not make you feel deprived or frustrated because it is so easy to follow. You do not even need to have a really strong determination because it is all a matter of choosing natural over artificial.

Is there such a thing as 'dirty' eating?

You are probably wondering if there is such a thing as 'dirty' eating or the opposite of clean eating. Clean eating does not literally mean eating foods that have less dirt. It means that you are choosing the best and healthiest food choices from different food groups in their most natural state. 'Dirty' eating is not the opposite of clean eating because there is no such thing as eating dirty. The opposite of clean eating is choosing the wrong food to eat and eating junk foods and processed foods that leave toxins in your body.

Clean eating also looks at the source of food. It should not come from large commercial manufacturers that use machines to process food. The foods that clean eaters usually use come from small farms that do not use chemicals and undergo processes. This is why clean eating is often associated with organic eating.

Chapter 2

Principles of Clean Eating

In every new diet program or plan, there are underlying principles that make up its foundation. These principles are the bases of the whole program or plan. Clean eating is not really a diet program but it also follows certain principles. Here are some of the basic principles of eating clean.

Eat Whole Foods

Whole foods are foods that are in their most natural state. This means that they have not been processed or tampered with in a factory or a laboratory. For example, the most natural state of an apple fruit is after you pick it directly from the tree. It becomes processed or tampered with when they extract juice from the fruit and add sweeteners and flavorings to produce ready-to-drink apple juice. On the other hand, homemade apple pies, apple marmalades, and apple cider are still good for clean eating because they are not processed in a factory and chemicals and artificial ingredients are not added. Whole foods come straight from the farm. Some examples include whole grains, fresh fruits and vegetables, unsalted nuts and seeds, and so on.

Avoid Processed Foods

Obviously, you should also avoid processed foods if clean eating involves eating only all-natural or whole foods. Processed foods have labels. You can see at the back of the food product that it has additional ingredients, preservatives, and other artificial substances to make the food last long and also to ensure that it tastes just like all the others. There are some foods that are processed in factories such as natural cheeses and whole grain pasta but these are not necessarily bad because they usually do not have artificial ingredients. The trick is to not buy any food item that has more than five ingredients or if the names of the ingredients are difficult to pronounce.

Do Not Use Refined Sugar

That fine white sugar may look cleaner than brown sugar but you should avoid this type of sugar because this has already been refined in the factory. Refined sugar has that sweet artificial taste which is so much different from the natural sweet taste of brown sugar. You should eliminate this from your diet because it only gives nothing but calories. To sweeten your food and drinks, you can use brown sugar or honey instead.

Combine Proteins, Carbs, and Good Fats

Some people who go on a diet make the mistake of removing one food group from their diet plan, such as carbohydrates, protein, or fat. This is not healthy because your body needs these nutrients. What you can do is to eat a balanced meal that has contains the right amount of protein, carbohydrate, and fats that your body needs. Combining these nutrients also make you feel more satisfied and full, which keeps you from snacking on junk food or eating more than what is necessary. This combination also gives enough fuel for your body to get you through the whole day.

Prepare your Own Meals

Instead of eating out, you should consider preparing your own meals at home. You should also consider packing your own lunch when you go to work. This is the best thing to do if you are planning to try clean eating because you know that the ingredients that you used to prepare the meal are natural and unprocessed. You should also avoid buying those ready-to-cook or instant meals in a box because these foods usually contain artificial ingredients. You can try some of the recipes that are included in this book.

Eat Smaller Meals

Instead of eating two or three large meals in a day, you should consider eating five to six smaller meals throughout the day to improve your metabolism and also to maintain that feeling of being full that will keep you from snacking on any food that you can find in the fridge or binge eating.

Avoid High Calorie Drinks

You should avoid high calorie drinks such as coffee or soft drinks because they add around 400 to 500 calories in a day, which is difficult to burn. Clean eating does not really require you to count your calories but it also does not mean that you can consume high calorie foods and drinks anytime you like. If you are thirst, you can drink water, unsweetened tea, or freshly squeezed fruit juice.

Chapter 3

Benefits of Clean Eating

Clean eating has a lot of benefits to your health. This is the reason why a lot of people want to try this way of eating. It is one of the key components of having a healthy lifestyle. Here are some of the more specific benefits of clean eating.

Improve Health and Wellbeing

Eating clean helps improve your health because you are eating all-natural food that does not have any artificial or chemical ingredients that are harmful to your health. Toxins from processed food cause diseases such as cancer, heart problems, and diabetes, to name a few. Clean eating also promotes a balanced diet because it encourages you to eat the right amount of nutrients. And if your body is getting all the nutrients that it needs, it will have a stronger immune system which protects your body against diseases. Your body will also feel lighter because you consume less meat plus you choose meat that has the best quality. Some people even completely forgo eating meat and get their protein requirements from other sources although this decision is all up to you. And because you are not eating meat, diseases that are caused by eating too much meat can also be prevented such as high blood pressure and stroke.

Aside from improving your physical health, eating clean also helps improve your mental health. This is because you are getting nutrients that your body needs which greatly improves your mood and feelings. It also helps prevent feelings of depression and anxiety.

Lose Weight

Clean eating also helps you lose weight because you are eating the right amount of food and the kinds of food that keep you feeling full. This is especially true if you are not eating a lot of meat because meat can contribute to weight gain. You do not need to try those expensive diet fads that become popular each year. You do not even need to make a lot of effort if you try clean eating. People who are not trying to lose weight shed extra fats and achieve their optimum weight without even trying after following the principles of clean eating. Clean eating also encourages you to eat five to six smaller meals in a day instead of three large meals. This method keeps you feeling full and satisfied throughout the day, which in turn keeps you away from snacks and sweets to satisfy your cravings and hunger pangs.

Boost Energy

People these days become exhausted easily because of their sedentary lifestyle. You often feel the slump after eating lunch. This can also be attributed to your unhealthy diet. If your diet consists mostly of refined sugar, you will have these dramatic energy spikes that tend to slow down in the afternoon making you feel lazy after lunch. If you change your diet and start eating clean, you will become more energized which in turn will make you more productive. And if you feel energetic, you will also be more inclined to exercise, which will further help you boost your energy, lose weight, and achieve good health.

Chapter 4

Tips for Getting Started

If this is your first time to try clean eating, you should learn some useful tips that will help you get started. These tips will make the transition from your old diet and eating habits to clean eating much smoother.

Define What Is Clean Eating For You

It has been mentioned in the previous chapters that the definition of clean eating varies from person to person. You need to have your own definition which will serve as your guide when buying food and preparing meals. The principles of clean eating are your basic guide but you can tweak them a little bit to better suit your personal needs and preferences. For example, one of the basic principles of clean eating is eating lots and lots of fruits and vegetables. If you like to add meat, you can do so because clean eating does not necessarily forbid you to eat meat. Just make sure that you are eating high quality lean meat.

Stock your Pantry with 'Clean' Foods

Now that you are starting this new way of eating, you should also do something about your pantry and your fridge which are most likely filled with processed food with artificial ingredients. Clean out your pantry and fridge by getting rid of food items that have artificial ingredients and that are obviously processed in factories. You can check the label and ingredients for this.

Once you are done cleaning out your pantry and fridge, you should now do your grocery shopping. Some may have a hard time coming up with a clean eating grocery list but it is actually simple. Just include lots of fresh fruits and vegetables and buy those products that have the word 'whole' in them such as whole wheat bread, whole wheat crackers, or whole pasta. Another keyword to look for is 'unsweetened' such as unsweetened almond milk, coconut milk, soy milk, and so on.

For food items that are difficult to find, such as a clean ketchup, you should consider making homemade ketchup using fresh tomatoes and other clean ingredients. It is important to prepare for the shopping trip especially if this is your first time by making a grocery list and doing a little research on food items that you can prepare yourself.

Give Yourself Time to Adjust

Transitioning from a lifestyle wherein you eat anything you like to a more disciplined eating habit like clean eating may be difficult for some, especially when they realize the amount of work involved in choosing the right kinds of food and preparing your own meals all the time. But once you get used to it and you started to reap the benefits of clean eating, everything will be so much easier. Just give yourself plenty of time to adjust. For example, you do not really have to give up all your favorite processed foods overnight such as pizza, cake, or doughnuts. You can still eat them while you are I the process of transitioning to clean eating. As you become accustomed to your new eating lifestyle, you can get rid of these processed foods one by one. You can find clean recipes of your favorite foods so that you can make them at home using clean ingredients.

These are the things that you need to know if you are planning to start a clean eating lifestyle. The next chapter includes some easy-to-make recipes that you can prepare for your whole family even when you are on the go.

Chapter 5

Simple and Easy Clean Eating Recipes

You will need some easy and simple recipes that you can whip up in just a few minutes if you are going to transition to a clean eating lifestyle. One great tip is to prepare your meals in big batches when you have free time and freeze small portions. This way, you and your family can just reheat the food whenever they need to eat. This will prevent you from eating out or eating just whatever is available. You might also want to invest in a cooler which you can pack with ice and take with you at the office or anywhere you go so that you can eat clean anytime, anywhere. You should also invest in a slow cooker where you can just leave the food that you are cooking while doing other things.

Here are some simple and quick clean eating recipes that are easy to prepare.

Cucumber and Tomato Salad

Ingredients:

- 2 medium-sized cucumbers, peeled and sliced thinly
- 2 cups cherry tomatoes, sliced in half
- ½ red onion, sliced thinly
- 1 tsp Dijon mustard
- 1 tbsp extra virgin olive oil
- 2 tbsp fresh dill
- 1 tsp honey (optional)
- Sea salt and pepper to taste

Procedure:

1. Combine cucumbers, tomatoes, and onion in one large salad bowl.

2. In a separate bowl, mix the remaining ingredients for the dressing using a whisk.

3. Pour the salad dressing into the vegetable mix. Toss to evenly coat the vegetables. Serve.

Roasted Salmon and Bok Choy

Ingredients:

- 2 8-oz salmon cut without skin
- 1 large bok choy, chopped
- ¼ cup white onion, chopped
- ¼ cup green peas
- ½ cup vegetable stock
- 4 tbsp butter
- 2 tbsp teriyaki sauce
- 2 tbsp olive oil
- ¼ tsp dried thyme
- 1 tsp sweet paprika
- Salt and pepper

Procedure:

1. Preheat oven to 375 degrees Fahrenheit.

2. Using a small brush, coat the salmon cuts with olive oil. Turn on the stove to medium heat and place a saucepan over the burner. Place the salmon on the saucepan, with the skin side facing down.

3. While one side of the salmon is cooking, use the same brush to apply teriyaki sauce on the top side of the salmon. Sprinkle a bit of salt, pepper, and paprika to season.

4. Put the salmon in the oven while it is still in the skillet and bake until the salmon is well cooked, which is around 15 minutes.

5. While waiting for the salmon to cook, steam the bok choy for about 10 mnuts or until they are properly cooked. You can also boil them, whichever you prefer.

6. Put a frying on the stove over medium heat and melt the butter. Add onion and cook for about five minutes or until translucent.

7. When the onion is cooked, add the veggie stock and the bok choy. Bring to a simmer.

8. Add the remaining ingredients which include the thyme and green peas. Sprinkle with salt and pepper to taste. Continue cooking until the liquid has evaporated, which is around 10 minutes.

9. Take out the salmon from the oven. Using aluminum foil, cover the skillet completely to allow the juices to evenly coat the salmon. Set this aside for about five minutes.

10. Put the bok choy on two separate plates and place the salmon on top. Serve while still hot.

Energy Booster Smoothie

Ingredients:

- 1 banana
- 1 cup raw oats
- 1 cup almonds
- 1 cup blue berries
- 1 tbsp chia seeds
- 1 tbsp ground flax
- 1 tbsp cocoa powder
- ½ cup plain greek yogurt
- 1 tbsp coconut oil
- A large drizzle of honey (the amount depends on how sweet you want it to be)
- A spoonful of homemade peanut butter
- Ice cubes

Procedure:

1. Put everything in a blender and blend until the mixture becomes thick and smooth, like a smoothie. Put in a pitcher and serve immediately.

2. This recipe includes a little bit of everything. The ingredients are quite flexible. You can substitute other clean ingredients if you do not have one or two of the ingredients above.

Blueberry Scones with Orange Zest

Ingredients:

- ½ cup frozen blueberries
- Zest of 1 orange
- 1 cup cashew flour
- 1 cup almond flour
- 1 cup coconut flour
- 1 tbsp hard coconut oil
- 1 ½ cups almond milk
- ¼ cup coconut sugar
- 2 tbsp baking powder
- a pinch of salt

Procedure:

1. Preheat oven to 400 degrees Fahrenheit. Get a baking sheet and line it with parchment paper.

2. In a large mixing bowl, combine the different kinds of flours, the baking powder, and salt and mix together using a spatula.

3. Cut the hardened coconut oil into small chunks using a fork and add this in your flour mixture. Mix together until the texture becomes crumbly. Add the orange zest and sugar and mix together using a fork.

4. Add the milk into the mixture and mix using a spatula.

5. Fold the blueberries into the mixture until they are evenly distributed throughout the dough.

6. Put the dough in your baking sheet lined with parchment paper and form a circle using your hands. The dough should be about 12 inches wide and an inch thick.

7. Once you are done shaping the dough, sprinkle the top with sugar.

8. You can use a knife to slice through the dough to make 8 scones. Do this as if you are slicing a pizza.

9. Bake the scones until the edges are brown and crisp, which is about 20 minutes, give or take a couple of minutes.

10. Once baked, take the scones out from the oven and set aside to cool.

11. You can separate the scones apart using a spatula or a knife before serving.

Slow Cooked Savory Soup

Ingredients:

- 1 large sweet potato, cubed
- 2 cups carrots, sliced
- 1 cup green beans
- 1 small onion, diced
- 1 clove garlic, minced
- ½ cup fresh cilantro, chopped
- 15 oz (2 cans) black beans in can, drained and rinsed
- 2 cups vegetable juice
- 2 cups vegetable broth
- ½ tsp black pepper
- ½ tsp red pepper flakes, crushed
- 1 tsp cumin
- 1 tsp chili powder
- Sea salt to taste

Procedure:

1. Put all the ingredients in a slow cooker. Cover the cooker with the lid and cook on low setting until the veggies are tender, which takes about 6 to 8 hours.

2. You can add about a teaspoon of cheese if you like.

3. You can also sauté the onion and garlic in olive oil before adding to slow cooker together with the other ingredients for a more subtle flavor.

4. You can also add about 2 cups of kale, coarsely chopped, at the last five minutes of cooking. Kale is also considered a superfood because of the amount of nutrients that it provides.

Turkey with White Bean Chili

Ingredients:

- 1 lb ground lean turkey
- 19 oz (1 can) white kidney beans, drained and rinsed
- 4 tsps chili powder
- 1 medium-sized onion, chopped
- 28 oz (1 can) whole tomatoes with juice, chopped
- 1 tbsp ground cumin
- ½ cup plain yogurt
- ½ cup water

Procedure:

1. Turn on the stove to medium heat and put a 12-inch skillet. Put the turkey on the skillet, adding salt for seasoning, and cook until the turkey is slightly browned, which is around 6 to 8 minutes. Continuously stir the turkey using a spoon to break it up into smaller pieces. Cook the onion in the same skillet for 4 minutes, and add cumin and chili powder. Cook some more for about a minute.

2. Add the beans, tomatoes with the juice, and water. Cook until the mixture is boiling. Reduce the heat to low and let it simmer without the cover for about 10 minutes. Serve the chili in bowls and top it with a spoonful of yogurt.

Quinoa Salad with Orange, Dates, and Asparagus

Ingredients:

For the salad:
- 1 cup raw quinoa
- ½ cup white onion, chopped
- I cup fresh orange sections
- 5 dates, pitted and chopped
- ½ lb asparagus slices, steamed and chilled
- ½ cup jalapeno pepper, diced
- ¼ cup pecans, chopped and toasted
- 2 tbsp red onion, minced
- 2 cups water
- 1 tsp olive oil
- ½ tsp sea salt

For the dressing:
- 2 tbsp lemon juice, freshly squeezed
- 1 garlic clove, minced
- 2 tbsps fresh mint, chopped
- 1 tbsp extra virgin olive oil
- ¼ tsp black pepper, freshly ground
- ¼ tsp sea salt
- Mint sprigs (optional)

Procedure:

1. For the salad: In a large non-stick skillet, heat the olive oil over medium heat. Sauté white onion for two minutes. Add quinoa and sauté for another 5 minutes. Add water and salt and bring the mixture to a boil. Once boiling, lower the heat and cover the skillet and let is simmer for 15 minutes. Turn off the heat and remove from the stove. Set aside for about 15 minutes to let the quinoa absorb the water. Put

the quinoa mixture in a large bowl and add the orange sections and the remaining ingredients. Mix gently.

2. For the dressing: Mix together all the ingredients, except the mint and mint sprigs, in a small bowl. Pour the dressing into the salad and gently toss until the dressing evenly coats the salad. Add the fresh mint and garnish with mint sprigs. Serve.

Black Bean Casserole

Ingredients:

- 15 oz (2 cans) black beans, drained and rinsed
- ½ cup vegetable broth
- 4 whole-wheat, low-sodium tortillas
- 1 cup shredded cheese
- 2 garlic cloves, minced
- 2 tbsp cilantro, chopped
- 12 oz unsweetened salsa
- ¼ tsp black pepper
- 1 tsp cumin
- 2 tbsp extra virgin olive oil
- Salt to taste

Procedure:

1. Preheat oven to 375 degrees Fahrenheit. Put skillet over medium heat and add olive oil. Saute garlic on the skillet before adding black beans and vegetable broth. Cook for three minutes. Add the spices such as cilantro, cumin, black pepper, and salt. Stir to evenly distribute the flavors.

2. Get an 8x8-inch casserole and spray with cooking spray. Put one tortilla on the dish, a quarter portion of the black bean mixture, a quarter portion of the salsa, and a quarter of cheese. Do the same steps until you have used up all the ingredients.

3. Once you are done layering the tortilla, black beans, salsa, and cheese, you should now cover the dish with aluminum foil. Put it in the oven and bake for about 20 minutes. You will know when it is cooked when the cheese becomes bubbly. Remove foil and put it back in the oven for another

8 to 10 minutes. Remove from the oven for the last time. You can add sour cream or Greek yogurt if you like.

Strawberry Cream Pie Parfaits

Ingredients:

- 1 ¼ lb fresh strawberries, sliced
- 1 cup whole-wheat flour
- 1 ½ cup ricotta cheese
- ¼ cup almond meal
- 3 tbsp raw honey, divided
- 2 tbsp safflower oil
- ¼ tsp sea salt
- 2 tbsp cold water

Procedure:

1. Preheat oven to 350 degrees F. spray an 8-inch square baking dish made of glass with cooking spray.

2. Combine almond meal, flour, and salt in a medium bowl using a whisk. Add safflower oil, honey, and cold water. Do not add these ingredients all at the same time. Be sure to stir the mixture until the ingredient is incorporated into the mixture before adding the next ingredient. The mixture will have a sandy texture, which is a little uneven.

3. Transfer the mixture into your baking dish and gently press with your fingers to ensure that the layer is even. Bake for about 21 to 24 minutes. Once the edges and bottom part are golden brown in color, take it out from the oven and let it cool.

4. Mix together honey and cheese in a bowl. You can use an electric mixer on high speed setting. Remove the crust from the baking sheet once it is cooled and place on a cutting board or any clean flat surface. Break the crust into bite-size pieces.

5. To assemble the parfait, you will need 6 parfait glasses. Divide the crust, strawberries, and cheese into six parts. Add your crust, cheese, and strawberries into the glass. Do this for all the other parfait glasses.

Crab Salad-Stuffed Eggs

Ingredients:

- 1 cup lump crabmeat
- 2 cups radishes, sliced thinly
- 8 large eggs
- 24 butter lettuce leaves
- 2 tbsp extra virgin olive oil
- 1 tbsp freshly squeezed lemon juice, divided
- 1 tsp dry mustard
- ¼ cup celery, finely chopped
- ¼ tsp ground black pepper
- 3 tbsps Greek yogurt
- ½ tsp salt, divided

Procedure:

1. In a large bowl, mix radishes, 1 tsp lemon juice, and salt. Cover with lid or plastic wrap and put it in the fridge for about 30 minutes.

2. Boil eggs in a medium saucepan. Be sure to cover the eggs with cold water. Once the eggs are boiling, reduce the heat and let it simmer for ten minutes. Turn off the stove and put the eggs in cold water to let them cool. Once the eggs are cool enough to hold, crack the egg shells and peel. If it is still a little too hot, you can peel the eggs under running water. After peeling the eggs, cut them in half vertically. Take out the egg yolks and put them in a sieve. You will need about 1 tbsp of yolks so set this aside.

3. In a medium bowl, combine the remaining lemon juice, ¼ teaspoon salt, pepper, and remaining egg yolks. Mix together using a whisk. Gradually add the oil while continuously stirring. Add the yogurt, crabmeat, mustard,

and celery. Gently stir until all the ingredients are well combined. Add salt and pepper to taste.

4. Create a fan using three lettuce leaves on each of the 8 plates. You should cut a very small part under the egg white to keep it steady. Add the crab filling into each egg white half. Each plate will have two egg whites. Add 1 tsp of egg yolk on top of the crap filling. Put the two egg white halves on one side of the plate and put sliced radish mixture on the other side. Do the same steps for all the remaining plates and ingredients.

Conclusion

Thank you again for purchasing this book!

I hope this book was able to help you to learn more about clean eating and how it can improve your health and well-being.

The next step is to start eating clean by following the guidelines that you have learned in this book. You should also try some of the quick and easy recipes included in the last chapter.

Finally, if you enjoyed this book, please take the time to share your thoughts and post a review on Amazon. It would be greatly appreciated!

I would love for you to share your experiences, stories and encouragements with me. My email address is emmarosekindle@gmail.com

In addition, please remember to check out our Facebook page in order to find other resources and upcoming promotions:

https://www.facebook.com/joypublishing

With sincere thanks,

Emma Rose

Preview Of "Paleo Diet Guide for Beginners: Over 50 Paleo Diet Recipes for Fast Weight Loss and Optimal Health"

Introduction

I want to thank you and congratulate you for purchasing the book, *"Paleo Diet Guide for Beginners: Over 50 Paleo Diet Recipes for Optimal Health and Fast Weight Loss"*.

This book contains everything you might need to know when it comes to getting started with the Paleo diet. It is provided in an easily digestible format that allows you to better absorb the information. There are no complicated explanations about how it works! You'll be given what you need straight up so you won't have to waste time trying to understand exactly what the diet is. Whether it's for your overall good health or to lose a few pounds, Paleo can certainly help you with it. To help you get started, we'll do the same and start you off with 50 of the best Paleo recipes that you can slowly but surely shift your everyday menu to.

It's never easy changing a diet. I often fall into self pity when I can no longer have the foods I enjoy. Either I feel sorry for myself or I get rebellious and binge and anything and everything. I always knew the value of eating healthy. I could just never bring myself to do it. It wasn't until I had a miscarriage that I got serious about my health. I have made drastic changes that others just don't understand. But the pay off is the weight I've lost and the better health I'm experiencing.

My hope for you is not to be on another "diet." This isn't a restriction diet like Atkins. The goal is to have a lifestyle change. Lifestyle changes are more sustainable and maintain weight loss long term compared to restriction diets. The change is hard to start but worth it when you commit. The trick is to get the momentum to start.

Thanks again for purchasing this book. I hope you enjoy reading it and eating the recipes from it!

With gratitude,

Emma Rose

Chapter 1 – What Is the Paleo Diet?

The Paleo Diet is known by many names such as the cavemen diet, stone age diet and hunter-gatherer diet, to name a few. The concept behind this diet follows that of the Paleolithic era before the development of agriculture. Essentially, you consume the same foods that the cavemen used to eat. The focus is on eating food closest to its natural, unprocessed state. The cavemen would gather their food from any source available whether it was wild animals, berries, vegetables, or fruits. As a result, they were strong, fit, and healthy for thousands of years.

This type of diet is still very young, less than fifty years only, but more in depth researches and studies are being conducted to increase the information and knowledge on this diet. The results of previous studies conducted on the Paleo diet reveal the improvement of health to the people involved. This is attributed to the fact that no processed foods and additives are included. The Paleo Diet is a diet that works with our genetics – before machinery and processing got involved. Foods that were not available during the Paleolithic time such as dairy products, salt, sugar and grains are not included in the preparation of the Paleo diet.

The modern diet predominately consumed in the Western world is full of refined foods, trans fats, salt and sugar. These ingredients are known to indirectly cause diseases such as hypertension, diabetes, strokes, obesity and other heart problems. The list goes on even further with the increase diagnosis of cancer, Parkinson's, Alzheimer's, depression and infertility. "What an extraordinary achievement for a civilization: to have developed the one diet that reliably makes its people sick!" (Michael Pollen, Food Rules: An Eater's Manual, Penguin Books 2009).

Foods included in the Paleo Diet

- Fruit

- Vegetables

- Lean Meat

- Seafood

- Nuts/Seeds

- Healthy Fats (eg. coconut, avocado, nuts and seeds, olive oil, grass fed butter)

Foods NOT included in the Paleo Diet

- Dairy

- Grain

- Processed Food

Why not grain?

You may be surprised to see that grains are not included in the Paleo Diet. We are accustomed to grains being a part of a balanced diet. However, our bodies are not designed to deal with the nutritional components of grains such as gluten, lectin, and phytates.

Gluten is a protein substance found in wheat, barley and rye. Many people are discovering that their bodies are gluten sensitive and are eliminating gluten from their diet. The most extreme case of gluten sensitivity is Celiac Disease. Individuals with this disease can pick up the minutest trace of gluten and react immediately.

Lectin binds to insulin receptors and can also cause leptin resistance.

Phytates cause minerals to become unavailable during digestion.

Check out the rest of "Paleo Diet Guide for Beginners: Over 50 Paleo Diet Recipes for Fast Weight Loss and Optimal Health" on Amazon.

Or go to: http://amzn.to/1jIJUFX

Detox Diet Guide

Lose Weight Quickly, Achieve Optimal Health and Feel Energized Through the 10 Day Detox

Emma Rose

Table of Contents

Introduction

I want to thank you and congratulate you for purchasing the book, *"Detox Diet Guide: Lose Weight Quickly, Achieve Optimal Health and Feel Energized Through the 10 Day Detox"*.

This book contains proven steps and strategies on how to not just simply flush out toxic substances from our bodies, but to also enhance the way our bodies naturally flush out those toxins.

It also contains other important information such as the most common toxins that are found in the environment that we unknowingly consume, the many ways our bodies naturally detoxify themselves, the things one must and must not do within the ten days of the detox diet, detoxification recipes that can be easily prepared, and some important reminders that must be taken before, during, and after the detox diet.

Thanks again for purchasing this book. I hope you enjoy it! Please take some time to stop by and LIKE our Facebook page:

https://www.facebook.com/joypublishing

With gratitude,

Emma Rose

Emma Rose

Chapter 1: Toxins and the Body

As the human body does its usual processes, some things need to be expelled. These are usually waste products made as a result of filtering out substances not needed by the body. There is a reason for the so-called "calls of nature" – which are peeing and releasing excrement.

But sometimes, those unwanted substances can build up in the organs and the bodily systems that comprise them. If there are too much of those substances, they will cause all sorts of harm to the overall bodily functions that can lead to various ailments.

The Top 10 List of Most Common Toxins

Human civilization evolves as a result of the desire of the people to live more comfortably and conveniently. But in the process of that evolution, it has unknowingly unleashed a cavalcade of impurities that do not just pollute the environment, but also the human body. Despite the many efforts by several government agencies and private individuals to thwart the sources of those impurities, there are traces of those impurities that still linger around. Those traces remain in the air, in the soil, in several bodies of water – and eventually, in the foods that humanity consumes.

According to Dr. Joseph Mercola, a well-known personality in the US wellness movement and owner and founder of Mercola.com (one of the most-trusted health websites), the ten most common toxic substances that are still prevalent in the environment to this day are the following:

1. Polychlorinated biphenyls, or PCBs, were commonly dumped by factories into nearby bodies of water. Due to their toxicity, PCBs were banned decades ago. However, traces of PCBs can still be found in those bodies of water since the toxic substances do not break down easily even after all those years. Fish that swim in those bodies of water still consume PCBs

unknowingly. As people still eat those fish, they will also ingest PCBs that will contribute to ailments such as cancer and brain defects in newborn babies.

2. Pesticides, while they do kill pests as their name says, are the major contributors of cancer. As farms still use synthetic pesticides such as weed killers, fungi killers, and insect killers; residues of those pesticides still remain in as much as 50 to 90 percent of US farm produce. Furthermore, there are bug sprays used to kill cockroaches and other unwanted insects in homes. Those bug sprays also contain the same carcinogenic substances as farm-focused pesticides. Besides cancer, pesticides also cause Parkinson's disease, miscarriage, nerve damage, birth defects, and getting in the way of nutrient absorption.

3. Fungal toxins not just come in the form of poisonous mushrooms. The most common of those fungal toxins is mould. Mould thrives in moist places such as bathrooms and kitchens; and can even sustain in vulnerable foods such as peanuts, wheat, and corn. One in three people are allergic to this fungal toxin. If left unchecked, mould causes cancer, heart disease, asthma, multiple sclerosis, and diabetes.

4. Phthalates are commonly found in plastic products and are responsible for softening them, making them easier to mold. They can seep into foodstuffs and drinks that are placed inside plastic food containers and plastic bottles. The result of ingesting too much phthalates is hormonal imbalance, since the substances resemble naturally-produced hormones. In children, phthalates can stunt their growth.

5. Volatile organic compounds, or VOCs, are commonly found in several household products such as air fresheners, cleaning fluids, mothballs, and varnishes. VOCs aid in air pollution and cause several sicknesses such as cancer, irritation of eyes and lungs, headaches, dizziness, and impaired memory.

6. Dioxins are some of the pollutants that are produced when something is burned, especially in massive quantities. As they

are released into the air, humans not just breathe in the dioxins. Livestock can also inhale those toxins and settle in their fats even after they are brought to the slaughterhouse to be made into meat. Dioxins cause cancer, stunted growth, reproductive system impairments, skin disorders such as acne, and slight damage to the liver.

7. Asbestos was a popular insulation material, but it was banned in the seventies due to its carcinogenic effects. Traces of asbestos can still be found in old homes that did not have their insulations replaced. Besides cancer, asbestos causes scarring on the lung tissue.

8. Toxic heavy metals such as lead, arsenic, and mercury can still be found in various objects such as cheaply-made toys, preserved wood, antiperspirants, and building materials. Once those metals are inhaled or ingested, they can cause cancer, brain and nerve disorders such as Alzheimer's disease, nausea, lesser amounts of red and white blood cells, and abnormal heartbeats.

9. Chloroform is a common chemical that is used to make other chemicals. It is prevalent in the air, in water, and in food. It can cause cancer, infertility, birth defects, headaches, dizziness, and damage to the liver and kidneys.

10. Chlorine is commonly found in water as it is used to purify it. Whether from the typical drinking water or from a swimming pool, too much of chlorine will cause all sorts of respiratory problems such as sore throat, accumulation of fluid in the lungs, and asthma.

Based on this list, many of those toxins in the environment are brought about by humanity's modern lifestyles. Before they do undue harm to the body, especially the dreaded cancer, they must be flushed out promptly.

Other Sources of Toxins

Besides the ten most common toxic substances, there are also other toxins that can be found in almost everything in the modern world. It is inevitable that one must intake those toxins unknowingly, one way or the other.

The two most popular vices, which are smoking and drinking, are the other major reasons for the body's toxicity. Both alcohol and nicotine have been proven many times by the scientific community to be not just toxic, but also addicting. Those two substances also alter the brain's functions. Other toxic substances include caffeine, empty sugars, and saturated fats. The latter two are especially notorious for being fat fodder since they cannot be processed into needed energy.

Many cosmetics today also contain toxic substances such as VOCs that can be absorbed into the skin. Some cosmetics producers have already taken steps in ridding their beauty products of those toxins.

Taking too many medications all at once can also cause the body to be laced with toxins, since they are not properly eliminated from the body. If the body feels too taxed from a cornucopia of meds, a consultation with the doctor will help.

There are also naturally-occurring toxins that are used by certain plants and animals as defense mechanisms against invaders. Snakes and jellyfish have highly deadly toxins and should not be consumed as food. A Japanese dish called *fugu* uses a type of blowfish that releases toxins which will certainly kill someone who eats an improperly-prepared version of the dish.

Processed foods, especially canned goods, are also a major source of toxins. While those foods contain preservatives that prolong their shelf lives, they unknowingly unleash a world of hurt on one who voraciously eats these. Needless to say, one must balance those foods out with naturally-grown foods.

Chapter 2: Why Must We Detoxify?

Detoxification is not just the simple flushing out of unwanted substances when the body cannot handle expelling them on its own. It is also the purging of impure thoughts in the mind that cause all sorts of decisions to inhale and ingest several toxins, whether knowingly or unknowingly, into the body. To ensure that an individual is rightfully clean in both body and mind, all sorts of unwanted things must be eliminated, especially in the detox diet.

The Body Does It Own Job...

The excretory system does its job of purging waste substances from the body via its two major processes: urination and release of excrement. Urination is obviously handled by the urinary system, while the release of excrement is handled by the lower parts of the digestive system.

The urinary system's main actor is the kidneys. The kidneys filter unwanted stuff such as ammonia, urea, uric acid, and excess salt and water from the blood as well as other bodily fluids. Those unwanted stuff then get to the bladder, which acts as a temporary storage. If the bladder gets full, the stuff gets expelled out of the urethra in the form of urine. Ammonia is a byproduct of the breakdown and usage of protein for the body's energy, while urea and uric acid are less toxic substances that result from the breakdown of ammonia.

The lower parts of the digestive system consist of the liver, the intestines, and the colon. The liver does its job of breaking down foreign substances so that the kidneys can have an easier job filtering them out as urine. The intestines and the colon facilitate the expelling of solid waste substances in the form of feces. The colon, in particular, absorbs trace minerals such as potassium and sends them to the bloodstream before they are included as feces that will be expelled by pooping.

Another natural detoxifier found in the human body is the lymphatic system. The lymphatic system contains lymph nodes that are scattered throughout the body but are interconnected. Those nodes provide the body with immunity, complementing the immune system, by filtering out unwelcome invaders such as bacteria, viruses, old red blood cells, and other toxic substances.

Other parts of the excretory system consist of the lungs and skin. The lungs expel excess water and carbon dioxide when someone breathes out. The skin kicks out excess water, salt, uric acid, and excess trace minerals in the form of sweat.

...But It Is Not Enough in the Modern Age

However, as demonstrated in the previous chapter, there are far too many substances that are deemed toxic in the wrong amounts. With humanity's modern lifestyles, the body does not know what to make of the increasing number of unwelcome invaders in its insides. These usually never get flushed out as urine and feces, but instead accumulate in the body fat.

As the invaders multiply and never get flushed out, they get in the way of the body's usual processes and will cause several problems such as depleted energy levels, unnatural weight gain, and various diseases that target the major body systems.

Another thing that is not helping the body in its natural detoxification process is the busy and hectic schedules people normally have. Because those people have no time to perform even mundane healthy tasks such as drinking adequate water, the body never gets its supply of natural detox assistants. Couple the lack of those assistants with stress and it will be a recipe for disaster.

Therefore, it is important that in this world of toxicity, people must amplify their bodily defenses against all sorts of foreign toxic substances by enhancing the many components of the excretory system such as the kidneys, the liver, the intestines, and the colon. With the contaminants out of the way, the body's natural healing processes also get their groove back. As the major

8

organ systems work hand-in-hand, the benefits that are felt in one particular system will spread towards the other systems.

In short, steeling the body and its functions, especially the excretory functions, is one of the first lines of defense against toxin-induced sicknesses. There will be a marked loss in weight, since the excessive fats as well as the toxins they contain are properly expelled. There will also be renewed liveliness since the bodily functions that have something to do with the intake and processing of energy sources are no longer clogged by invasive toxins.

Why the Mind Is Also Important in Detoxification

The decisions a person makes, no matter how small they are, can contribute to huge consequences. For example, if one decides to commute to a bar, he or she gets all sorts of toxins in the process – airborne impurities from urban roads, food additives from the snacks he or she eats while commuting, nicotine and other chemicals from tobacco smoke generated by smokers inside and outside the bar, and alcohol from the hard drinks he or she consumes while in the bar.

Therefore, it is important that a person must think thoroughly and deeply before settling on a decision that will make him or her take in all those unwanted toxins along the way. Yes, this may turn him or her into a control freak, but there are also decisions that will endow him or her with long-term benefits. Remember, detoxification starts in the mind. The decisions that lead to the unknowing intake of toxins must be sorted out and eliminated from the usual routines first.

Chapter 3: The Crucial Ten Days

There are several forms of detoxification, and they more often than not involve ingesting special liquids and solids, cleansing the colon, foot baths and foot pads, spas and saunas, and fasting. But they also cost money, are always focused on the short-term effects, and may not deliver the detoxification results one desires. The best form of the detox diet must involve getting rid of major sources of toxins, ingesting more of the substances that will greatly assist the body's natural detoxification processes, never integrating any form of starvation or elimination of a major food group from the diet, and clearing the mind of impure thoughts that lead to impure actions. This way, the diet will grant long-term effects of well-being. As a beneficial consequence, this diet will cost little to no money, except for the money to be spent on detoxifying foods and drinks.

The ten days this detox diet contains are important to ensure natural weight loss and general well-being. And even after the diet period ends, some good habits contained in this diet, particularly the continued eating of healthy foods, must still be kept. This is to ensure that the person undergoing this diet will transition into a healthy lifestyle.

Preparing for the Diet

One important thing to do when undergoing this diet, or any other diet for that matter, is to not rush in immediately. A crash diet will have nasty consequences such as abrupt changing of body patterns that lead to all sorts of ailments as well as retention of the weight one lost during the diet routine. Therefore, one must start slow and transition into the diet carefully.

Not rushing in also applies to the chewing of food. The body needs some time to digest the food. Never treat the ten days of the diet like some kind of work deadline.

The usual vice-based sources of toxins, which are tobacco and alcohol, must be eliminated first. While dealing with the withdrawal effects of both of those substances may be difficult, timely help from a doctor who has a specialization in several types of addictions and substance abuse will lessen the difficulty.

In the three days before the actual start of the diet, rid the pantry and fridge of tempting foodstuffs that are loaded with empty calories. These include sweets and most forms of processed foods and fast food. At the same time, steadily increase the intake of fruits and vegetables – *especially organic ones*. As much as possible, turn the veggies into freshly-prepared salads and/or lightly steam them. As for the fruits, eat them raw and/or turn them into natural juices.

Since pesticide residue in fruits and vegetables is inevitable, the use of fruit and vegetable washes must be prioritized.

The intake of caffeine must be slowly and surely reduced to prevent withdrawal symptoms such as headaches. Switching to decaf coffee and low-caffeine teas such as green tea will help, as is the trick of diluting regular coffee and tea in huge amounts of water.

And speaking of water, the time-tested advice of eight to ten glasses of water a day will especially help the detox diet become successful. Drink it throughout the ten days of the diet.

Aromatherapy using essential oils is helpful, as this therapy helps to calm the mind in order for it to prepare for the rigors of the critical ten days.

Finally, before embarking on the detox diet itself, please consult a registered dietician who can recommend the detoxifying foods to be eaten based on your genetic makeup. Furthermore, *do not stop* taking prescribed medicine, as discontinuing medications can have devastating effects on the body. Diets are not meant to be one-man shows, especially if the individual still has to learn much about the intricacies of diet programs like this.

Eat and Drink Them

With the transition phase over, it is time to actually start the detox diet. Here is a comprehensive list of foods and drinks that must be ingested during the ten crucial days of the diet.

1. Organic fruits and vegetables are the main focus of the detox diet. It does not matter what the size or type of fruit or vegetable one will be consuming – as long as it is free of pesticides and synthetic fertilizers and is grown using age-old farming techniques, it certainly counts. Eat a good variety of fruits and vegetables to round out all the necessary nutrients.

2. Brown rice is much healthier compared to the typical white rice. As white rice is a result of the milling process, brown rice retains some nutrients that are usually lost during milling. This type of rice is also a rich source of fiber, which will aid in flushing the toxins out via the intestines and the colon.

3. Herbs are permissible, since they are also plants. Use them to flavor the dishes as well as utilize them for aromatherapy. Herbal teas are also a-OK, since they do not contain caffeine at all. As with fruits and vegetables, herbs must not have traces of anything toxic.

4. Whole-grain products, much like brown rice, do not undergo the nutrient-losing milling process. They are also rich sources of fiber. Whole-grain products include whole wheat bread, bran, and rolled oats.

5. Seaweeds such as kelp and *nori* wrappers used for sushi are also plant-based. They can also be consumed the same way as typical veggies do.

6. Beans such as green peas, chick peas, lentils, kidney beans, and black beans are permitted.

7. One can go nuts with nuts and seeds. Allowable things include almonds, cashews, walnuts, watermelon seeds, pumpkin

seeds, sunflower seeds, and sesame seeds. As a general rule, pick only raw, unsalted nuts and seeds.

8. Coconuts, while they are not actually nuts, are also allowed. There are several coconut-based consumables such as coconut water and coconut oil. One can also eat fresh coconut meat straight from the source.

9. Plant-based oils are encouraged. Olive oil, especially the extra virgin kind, is highly recommended.

10. Round out the protein-based nutrition with plant-based protein sources such as soy. Soy milk and tofu are easily-acquired sources of plant-based protein.

11. All sorts of edible mushrooms are permitted. Portobello and shiitake mushrooms can act as good substitutes for meat.

12. Natural sweeteners such as raw honey and natural maple syrup are permitted.

13. Besides herbs, other natural condiments that are tolerable include apple cider vinegar, sea salt, and mustard.

14. If there is still a desire to eat meat and get adequate protein, go with lean meats such as fish and organic chicken. Eggs are also on the list, as long as they are organic.

Never Eat and Drink Them

Meanwhile, these are the foods and drinks to avoid during the detox diet phase.

1. In general, non-lean types of red meat are off-limits. Canned meat is especially forbidden.

2. All forms of processed foods containing all sorts of additives and preservatives are out of the question. On a related note, artificial sweeteners and processed condiments are also out.

3. Typical white sugar and brown sugar are verboten, as well as high-fructose syrups.

4. Corn must be avoided as it is acid-forming. The acid in question is uric acid. Furthermore, the corn kernels that are indigestible will make bathroom breaks more excruciating.

5. While nuts are OK, peanuts and peanut butter are usually excluded.

6. Milk is normally not allowed, but half a cup of yogurt containing good bacteria per day is an exception to that.

7. Caffeine is another typical forbidden substance.

8. Shortening and margarine are inadmissible.

9. While fish is OK, other seafoods are not.

Other Cleansing Procedures

There are many variations of the detox diet, but the one being presented in this book will not involve complicated doohickeys and specialized food and drinks to amplify the detoxification effect. Here are some things one can also do during the ten days of the diet.

With all the conveniences of Internet-based connectivity, sometimes too much is too much. Dedicate one of the ten days, or even all ten days, to a temporary break from technology. Put away the smartphone or tablet, avoid touching the computer, and never be tempted to go online just about anywhere. Take the time off from technology to visit someplace serene, like a retreat house. This technology break will clear the mind of all sorts of burdening thoughts that may poison one's thinking the same way that bodily toxins do.

Take some time off to scrape the tongue. Tongue scraping is a practice in ayurvedic medicine, or ancient Hindu medicine, where all the impurities built up on the tongue are removed. Tongue scrapers can be bought for cheap at drug store.

Try to write all the stored thoughts and feelings, even negative ones, into a diary or notebook. Releasing all the stored strong emotions to a diary or notebook has a cathartic effect, since keeping those emotions locked away will eventually take the toll on one's health.

Another mind-cleansing procedure one can do during the ten days is meditation. Meditation also helps clear the mind of toxic thoughts that lead to stress, which then slows down the liver's detoxification process. Yoga is especially helpful as a meditation tool. You may also augment your meditation by doing deep breathing exercises or visualizing relaxing images such as watching the sunset at the beach.

Get enough dosages of vitamin C. While the vitamin is better known for boosting immunity, it also helps the body with the production of glutathione. Glutathione may be better known as a skin rejuvenating agent, but it also exists in the liver as a detoxification aid. Citrus fruits are the best-known sources of vitamin C.

Enhance blood circulation, since poor blood circulation will hamper the flushing out of impurities from the blood. Exercise is a guaranteed way to get that blood pumping.

Keep in mind that not all bacteria are bad. Good bacteria mostly reside in the intestines, aiding in digestion and preventing bad bacteria from releasing toxins that can be deployed in the bloodstream. Help the good bacteria by taking probiotic drinks.

Chapter 4: Detoxification Recipes

Breakfast Recipes

Gut-Busting Oatmeal Bowl

Ingredients:

- 1-2 cups oatmeal

- 1-2 cups water or nut milk

- A mixture of fresh berries and fresh fruits, all sliced

Procedure:

1. Prepare the oatmeal as indicated in the packaging.

2. While hot, pour the berries and fruits onto the prepared oatmeal, and mix.

Berry Blast Smoothie

Ingredients:

- 1-2 cups mixed fresh berries
- 1-2 cups protein powder
- 1-2 cups ice cubes

Procedure:

1. Throw all the ingredients into a blender, and hit puree.
2. Serve the smoothie in a tall glass.

Lunch Recipes

Veggie Cavalcade Salad with Tofu

Ingredients:

- 6-8 pieces of any whole vegetable (for greens, an amount of at least five leaves equals one whole piece)

- 1-2 pieces tofu, diced

- 4-5 teaspoons extra virgin olive oil

- 2 teaspoons fresh lemon juice

- 1 teaspoon freshly-chopped herbs of choice

Procedure:

1. Fry the tofu in 2-3 teaspoons olive oil until slightly browned. Set aside.

2. Slice and/or dice the vegetables into reasonably-sized pieces. Leave the greens untouched.

3. Pour all the vegetables and the tofu into a bowl. Mix completely.

4. Combine 2 teaspoons olive oil, the lemon juice, and the herbs to make the dressing.

5. Pour the dressing all over the salad. Mix completely.

Special Omelet Rice

Ingredients:

- 3-5 organic eggs
- Fresh or dried herbs (any variety), to taste
- 2-3 teaspoons extra virgin olive oil
- 1-2 cups cooked brown rice

Procedure:

1. Beat the eggs into a scramble while adding the herbs.
2. Pour the olive oil into a heated pan. Wait until the oil is hot.
3. Pour the egg and herb mixture until the omelet is formed. Turn over to ensure proper cooking.
4. Once the omelet is out of the pan, place the brown rice inside it. Make sure the omelet wraps around the rice.
5. Serve hot with mustard.

Dinner Recipes

The Steamed Medley

Ingredients:

- 1 slice salmon

- 5-10 pieces broccoli and asparagus (can be of any combination)

- 1/4 cup fresh lemon juice

- Fresh or dried herbs (any variety), to taste

Procedure:

1. In a steamer or a rice cooker with a steaming basket, arrange the salmon slice and the broccoli and asparagus pieces so that the steam will be evenly distributed.

2. Sprinkle the salmon and the vegetables with the lemon juice and fresh herbs.

3. Begin steaming the salmon and the vegetables. Seven to ten minutes is enough for the lemon and the herbs to seep into the steamed content.

4. Serve hot.

Glorified Bunch of Small Potatoes

Ingredients:

- 6 ounces small potatoes

- 4 tablespoons extra virgin olive oil

- Any natural condiment of choice

Procedure:

1. Gently simmer the potatoes in water for 5-10 minutes. Drain them off afterwards. Retain the peels beforehand.

2. Heat the olive oil in a roasting tin, but not to burning levels.

3. Roast every side of the potatoes until crisp and golden brown. This will take at most 45 minutes.

4. Serve hot with the condiment of choice.

Snack and Drink Recipes

Veggie Brown Rice Sushi

Ingredients:

- 1 cup cooked brown rice

- 1 *nori* wrapper

- Any sliced or diced vegetable that can fit inside the sushi

Procedure:

1. Mold the brown rice into any shape, whether in a tube form or rolled into a ball. The important thing is that the vegetable must fit inside the sushi.

2. Wrap the *nori* wrapper around the formed brown rice.

3. Repeat steps 1 and 2 for any remaining amounts of vegetables, brown rice, and the *nori* wrapper.

Stretched Herbal Iced Tea

Ingredients:

- 1 bag herbal tea (any kind)

- 1 citrus fruit of choice (e.g. lemon or orange)

- 1 cup briskly-boiled water

- 2-3 cups lukewarm water

- Several ice cubes

- Honey, to taste

Procedure:

1. Depending on the strength of the resultant tea, submerge one teabag into briskly-boiled water.

2. Meanwhile, cut the citrus fruit of choice into slices that can be fit inside a glass.

3. Place the fruit slices into a tall glass that can accommodate at least five cups.

4. Carefully pour both the brewed tea and the lukewarm water into the tall glass at a distance of at least 12 inches from the glass. This is where the "stretched" part comes from, and one must avoid spills during the stretching process.

5. Add some dollops of honey based on the preferred amount of sweetness.

6. Finally, add the ice cubes.

Fruity Shaved Ice

Ingredients:

- 1-2 cups shaved ice

- 1/2-1 cup natural unsweetened fruit juice of any kind

Procedure:

1. Place the shaved ice in either a wide glass or a bowl.

2. Pour the unsweetened fruit juice on top of the shaved ice, and enjoy.

Note: One can replace shaved ice with shaved or crushed frozen fruit.

Chapter 5: Some Friendly Reminders

As with every other diet program on the planet, care, precise planning, patience, and perseverance must be taken to heart when undergoing the detoxification diet. Even in a short period like ten days, many things will happen. To ensure that the detox diet will become a success that will beget many more successes in the realm of the healthy lifestyle, keep the following friendly reminders in mind.

Do Not Starve

Other detox diets recommend taking only the formulas they sell themselves. Indeed, they may contain needed plant-based nourishment needed for detoxification, but the makers of those diets often forget that an imbalanced diet that is lacking in calories will prove detrimental to the body. Not only will the energy levels be depleted, but the metabolism process will also be slowed down. One unpleasant aftereffect is the tendency to eat more, especially unhealthy foods, once the diet period is over. This will make natural weight loss almost unachievable. Even worse, the lack of micronutrients in these other detox diets will lead to malnutrition that is based on micronutrient deficiency, which opens yet another floodgate of diseases. Other nasty effects of other detox crash diets include muscle degeneration, since the muscles have no source of energy to turn to, and an imbalance in blood sugar levels.

Hence, this detox diet espouses the idea that *forced starvation is absolutely prohibited.* Just eat the recommended foods at will and in good, moderated amounts.

Expect to Pee (and Poop and Sweat) a Lot

Since the detox diet enhances the body's natural detox functions, expect one undergoing the diet to pee a lot. Water, in particular, helps in flushing out toxins.

Excessive peeing not just happens when the detox diet goes overboard. Excessive sweating also happens, as well as the resultant excrement being too liquid and nasty-smelling. Peeing, pooping, and sweating too much can lead to dehydration if the amount of fluids being taken is not immediately replenished.

Dehydration is not just the depletion of the body's water, but is also the disrupted balance of fluids and electrolytes that can lead to ailments such as gastrointestinal distress, headaches, fatigue, irritability, skin irritations, circulatory problems, kidney failure, and heat stroke. Death also awaits one who is severely dehydrated.

To counteract dehydration, do not depend on fluids and fluids alone, unlike what some detox diets emphasize. Be well-balanced in both solids and liquids to avoid lost hours as a result of abnormally frequent trips to the bathroom.

Want a Colonic? No Thanks

Another form of the detox therapy involves cleansing the colon and intestines of toxins that may be released into the bloodstream. However, as demonstrated in the third chapter, there are beneficial bacteria that reside in the colon and intestines. If those bacteria are flushed out, the normal digestive process will be hampered, and the bad bacteria will have a good time releasing more toxins since their rivals are gone. The flushing out of good bacteria also results from the detox diet going beyond the recommended ten days.

Another bad effect of colon cleansing is dehydration, for the same reasons demonstrated in the previous section. Trace minerals such as potassium are also lost during the cleansing process, which contributes to dehydration. Other side effects of colon cleansing include nausea and vomiting.

Diet as an End to the Means, Not a Means to the End

People who want the figures of their dreams often forget that dieting is not really meant to immediately shed unwanted pounds. Dieting is truly meant for improved nourishment and nutrition. The notions of shedding that slab or beer belly in preparation for an event like showing off in a bikini should be disposed of. A proper mindset must be established first when doing the detox diet or any other diet for that matter.

As stated before, the detox diet being demonstrated in this book should be a transitional phase to a healthier lifestyle. Thinking in the long term when dieting is certainly better than thinking in the short term. One should remember that dieting must be an end to unhealthy habits and not a means to end that "awful" figure.

Conclusion

Thank you again for purchasing *"Detox Diet Guide: Lose Weight Quickly, Achieve Optimal Health and Feel Energized Through the 10 Day Detox"*!

I hope this book was able to help you to understand the ins and outs of the detox diet and why it is important to achieve a major change in only a short time.

Are you ready for the change? Tony Robbins says in order to create effective change, you need to start by being disgusted with where you are at. Are you disgusted with your health or body? Is it an ABSOLUTE MUST to change...not another moment? You need to feel the pain of where you are at to get the urgency to change and manifest the momentum to take action.

The next step is to consult your doctor or dietician before embarking on such a diet. And once you are given the final OK, you can then consult various more detoxification recipes based on the comprehensive list of allowable foods and drinks in this book. The recipes given in this book is just a starting point.

Finally, if you enjoyed this book, please take the time to share your thoughts and post a review on Amazon. It would be greatly appreciated!

I would love for you to share your experiences, stories and encouragements with me. My email address is

emmarosekindle@gmail.com

In addition, please remember to check out our Facebook page in order to find other resources and upcoming promotions:

https://www.facebook.com/joypublishing

With sincere thanks,

Emma Rose

Preview of "Raw Food Diet Guide: Lose Weight Quickly, Achieve Optimal Health and Feel Energized with the Raw Food Diet and Raw Food Recipes"

Chapter 1

An Overview of the Raw Food Diet

The concept of the raw food diet is simple – cooking diminishes the nutritional value of food. Even though most of the food items in the diet are consumed while it is raw, heating is acceptable provided that the temperature stays between the range of 104 to 118°F or below.

Since cooking is perceived to kill off enzymes naturally found in food, raw food practitioners choose to avoid cooked food. As a matter of fact, overconsumption of cooked food forces the body to work overtime in order to produce more enzymes to support normal bodily functions. In the long run, the lack of enzymes can instigate a lot of problems involving a person's health, particularly accelerated aging, nutrient deficiency, weight gain and digestive problems.

Going raw can prove to be challenging, especially for those that are just starting out. It takes a lot of discipline to stick to the principles of the diet. Moreover, extra effort is required mentally and physically. When it comes to preparing your daily raw meals, your options are limited. Here are some of the procedures you may apply when organizing your meal plan:

- *Germination* – this is the process of soaking in water for a certain period of time. The recommended amount of time differs from one person to another but for raw foodists, the safest bet is to soak overnight.

- *Sprouting* – this comes after germination. After the beans, legumes or seeds are soaked, they may then be sprouted. Items should be left at room temperature until a sprout comes out of it. These sprouts may then be used for preparing food but should be rinsed and drained thoroughly beforehand.

- *Blending* – involves the use of a blender or food processor in order to create sauces, smoothies, or soup among others.

- *Dehydrating* – employs an equipment known as a dehydrator, which simulates sun drying. Common products of dehydrators are crackers, croutons, raisins, fruit leathers, sundried tomatoes, breads and kale chips.

- *Pickling* – a method of preserving food by marinating in a brine.

- *Juicing* – the process of extracting of vitamins, minerals and natural juices from plant tissues, particularly raw fruits and vegetables.

- *Fermentation* – process of converting sugar to carbon dioxide through the use of yeast.

Now that you know what procedures are available to you when preparing your raw meals, the next thing to know is which particular equipment/s you need to use. Below are some of the staple equipment that can be seen in every raw foodist's kitchen:

34

- *Dehydrator*—it is an enclosed container that has heating elements that can warm at low temperatures. It has a fan that blows warm air onto the food.

- *Spiral Slicer* – slices vegetables into spiral shapes

- *Thermometer* – to ensure that temperature stays below 118°F when heating food.

- *Trays* – for soaking and sprouting beans, legumes or seeds

- *Sprouters* or *mason jars*

- *Food processor*

- *Blender*

- *Juicer*

Check out the rest of "Raw Food Diet Guide: Lose Weight Quickly, Achieve Optimal Health and Feel Energized with the Raw Food Diet and Raw Food Recipes" on Amazon

Or go to: http://amzn.to/1xt93sY

Check Out My Other Books

Below you'll find some of my other books also available on Amazon and Kindle. Search for these titles on the Amazon website to find them.

Paleo Free Diet Guide for Beginners: Over 50 Paleo Free Recipes for Optimal Health & Fast Weight Loss

Paleo Desserts: Satisfy Your Sweet Tooth With Over 100 Quick & Easy Paleo Dessert Recipes & Paleo Baking Recipes

Raw Food Diet Guide: Lose Weight Quickly, Achieve Optimal Health & Feel Energized with the Raw Food Diet & Raw Food Recipes

Clean Eating Guide: Lose Weight Quickly, Achieve Optimal Health & Feel Energized with Clean Eating For Busy Families & Clean Eating Recipes

Alkaline Diet Guide: Lose Weight Quickly, Achieve Optimal Health & Feel Energized with the Alkaline Diet & Alkaline Recipes

Coconut Flour Recipes for Optimal Health & Quick Weight Loss: Gluten Free Recipes for Celiac Disease, Gluten Sensitivities & Paleo Free Diets

Almond Flour Recipes for Optimal Health & Quick Weight Loss: Gluten Free Recipes for Celiac Disease, Gluten Sensitivities & Paleo Free Diets

Wheat Free Diet for Beginners: Lose Weight Quickly, Achieve Optimal Health & Feel Energized with Gluten Free Recipes for Celiac Disease, Gluten Sensitivities & Paleo Free Diets

Detox Diet Guide: Lose Weight Quickly, Achieve Optimal Health & Feel Energized Through the 10 Day Detox

Sugar Detox Guide for Beginners: Lose Weight Quickly, Achieve Optimal Health, Feel Energized & Eliminate Sugar Cravings Naturally

Ketogenic Diet Guide for Beginners: How to Achieve Rapid Weight Loss, Optimal Health & Unstoppable Energy with Ketogenic Diet Recipes

Anti Inflammatory Diet for Beginners: Lose Weight Fast, Optimize Health, Slow Aging, Fight Inflammation, Conquer Pain & Increase Energy with the Anti Inflammation Diet Recipes

One Last Thing...

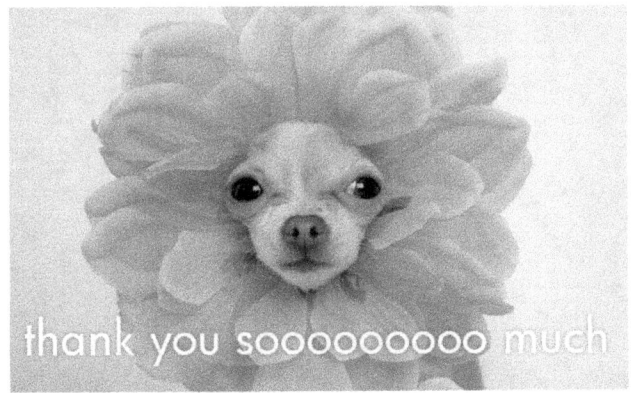

If you believe that this book is worth sharing, would you please take the time to let others know how it affected your life? If it turns out to make a difference in the lives of others, they will be forever grateful to you, as will I.